The Blue Jean Diet

Stop Dieting and Gain Your Ideal Figure

Jil Jennewein

Table Of Contents:

Chapter One:

Is Food Your Friend Or Foe?

"There is nothing either good nor bad, but thinking makes
it so."
William Shakespeare

How many of you reading this have tried every single diet you can think of, and you are still right back at square one needing to lose weight? You still look in the mirror and do not see a reflection of the real you, your inner you, looking back at you. You still can look in the mirror and say "I wish I looked better, thinner, healthier. I wish I looked like I used to." Well if that is you, if you are like me it isn't that you can't lose the weight. It is keeping off the weight once you have lost it that seems to elude you. I know. I've been there! I too have tried every diet in the library in order to lose weight with no long-term success. I tried the low carbohydrate, high protein diet. There is the grapefruit diet, the Hollywood liquid diet, fasting, Slimfast, Fit for Life and the food combination diet. Everyone has one! Reliv has shakes and bars. Usana has shakes and bars. Herbalife has shakes and bars. Shakes and bars. Yum!

I'm not saying that these diets don't work to lose weight. I mean, anyone can lose weight if you only eat 500 calories

a day. If you can keep yourself disciplined and

on a regiment to eating exactly what foods they say you

can eat, when they say you can eat them, you are most

definitely going to lose some weight. Everyone has got

a program to help you lose your weight. Richard Simmons

and Weight Watchers for instance. The list goes on and on.

They will help you count your calories or

carbs, and chart your food intake. They have notebooks

and special colored tabs and pens to help you to monitor

and keep track of fats and carbohydrates.

Everything you need to keep you on your regime. Regime.

Sounds like fun doesn't it? Just another system of rules

you are supposed to follow in order to get it right.

And if you get it right you get the promised result.

Well, supposedly. It feels so militant to me. Count two,

three, four, measure, two, three, four. I don't know about

you, but I want to enjoy my life, and my food. I don't want

to make eating just another set of rules I have to live by in order to look and feel good. No wonder we are an overweight society. Food is NOT the enemy. Food is to be enjoyed. How can anyone of us look at a well-cooked meal and say "I am NOT supposed to enjoy that." Whether it is steak, or a potato or a protein or a carbohydrate; how can we truly believe that we are not supposed to enjoy our food? Not just the aroma as it cooks, but eating it! Let alone chocolate mousse. No, no! That is bad! "I'm not supposed to enjoy this."

I admit, I have lost weight with the help of many of these diets. For years after giving birth to twin boys I struggled with losing the last 15 pounds that would put me at my ideal weight. I probably lost and gained hundreds of pounds over the course of eight years. I was so frustrated and felt such despair. I thought nothing was going to work for me. I joined Spa 80 for women. I would starve myself and lose 15-20 pounds on one of the many diets. But I could not for the life of me figure out how to keep it off. I didn't know how to continually, for the rest of my life, eat only "one sensible meal", and a shake or a bar for the other twomeals.

I don't know about you, but it was never enough for me to eat only chicken, fish, beef, cheese, eggs, nuts and lettuce. Or bars and shakes! How many bars and shakes can one person stomach in one life time? It just was not satisfying enough for a passionate food lover like me. I want to EAT! I want to eat ice cream and I want to eat it regularly. I love my toast and my cereal and pasta with white sauce or marinara sauce. I want it all! As long as I am alive I want to enjoy life. Life and all that it has to offer me including the simple pleasure of a great meal. I intend on enjoying food and my body feeling good all of the days of my life.

Chapter 2

You Are What You Think You Are

"Ninety-nine percent of who you are is invisible and untouchable." R. Buckminster Fuller

So, we know we can lose the weight. That is not the problem. We have lost it before and we can lose it again. And when we do, we are on the top of the world and the peak of our game and we feel great! For a couple of days or weeks you fit into all of your old cloths that you've waited so long to wear and you probably bought a couple nice outfits too. And then what happened?

Was it the six week run between Thanksgiving and Christmas with all of the dinner parties and 5 coarse meals? Was it the 7-day cruise you took with your sweetie with free food morning, noon and night that snuck up on you? What happened? Why couldn't you keep it off?

Well if the truth be known, I lost those 15 pounds immediately after delivering the twins. I went on the low carbohydrate, high protein diet. I was disciplined and regimented and motivated to get back into my cloths. And I did! The boys probably weren't a month old and I was back in my wardrobe again. I was so proud of myself and so was my husband. But then what happened?

Oh yes, the divorce. Stress of raising the twins alone. Fear, and lack of focus.

I had more important things to worry about than a waistline. I was feeling low and I looked to comfort foods. I just caved in! I couldn't keep eating fish and eggs. I gave into my body's natural cravings and urges. For eight years I hung onto those extra pounds after that and did the yo-yo dieting.

The more I focused on the food and the dieting and that I wasn't supposed to eat this or that; and if I could only eliminate certain foods I wouldn't have a problem; well focusing on trying to eliminate food, made food, a problem. The more I focused on my thick waistline being a problem, the more it was a problem. The more I focused on not exercising to burn calories as the problem, it was the problem. I actually gained weight while dieting and exercising. Now how on earth does that happen? Well, as I toned and built muscle while exercising, my thighs got bigger and since muscle weighs more than fat I had gained another 5-10 pounds. Now I was a solid over weight woman. Some would say that I was healthier and eating better, but all I knew was that I did not look my best. I did not look into the mirror and see a reflection of the spirit I knew I was inside. Therefore I did not feel my best either. I wasn't happy with the picture at all.

After trying everything for 8 years and losing and gaining and always ending up at square one, having changed nothing, I gave up! That's it! I just gave up! I threw away the diet books and the calorie counters and the food scales and the morning scale. (I suggest you do the same). The weight began to come off. I began to set myself free. Food became my friend and so did my body.

Set yourself free! Step one; throw away the diet books and the calorie counters. Release yourself from ever thinking about counting anything having to do with food again. Food is to be enjoyed and to nourish your body. That's it! Secondly, throw or give away your scales. All of them. Never look outside of yourself again for an indication of how your body looks and feels. Numbers do not matter. If you are worried about the number that the scale will reflect back to you each morning then you are still keeping your focus on the weight and off of how you feel.

If we have to weigh 125 in order to be happy and feel good, then every time you eat Christmas dinner or splurge a little you will get on the scale the next morning and panic. You will be up five pounds and all the old tapes will begin to play. All of your fears about gaining more weight if you eat anything today, or having to lose the weight and how hard that is, will kick in. If your belief is that you have to be a size 6 in order to be happy, then what happens when the department store you are shopping at makes their sizes small and you can't fit in a size 6? Their cloths are telling you that you are a size 8. This could be a problem if you are fixated on numbers and sizes. Numbers mean nothing and reflect no pertinent information back to you anymore.

My weight fluctuates between 5 pounds over or under my

Ideal weight all the time. And I have no idea, other than sometimes my cloths are loose and sometimes they feel a bit snug. And I have from size 4's to size 9 juniors in my closet. My natural size is about a 6, and I am guessing that I weigh about 125 pounds. But I really have no idea. I have not weighed myself in years. Even when I go in for a physical, I turn my head and I will tell the nurse that I "do not want to know. Don't tell me." Why? Because I know that if she says 135 I will freak out! When in fact I was having a great day and feeling great and thinking that I looked good too. And who is to say that her scale is right anyhow? Scales vary. I just do not let anything outside of myself tell me how I look or how I feel. I do not ask my boyfriend or my mother or best friend "how do I look?" I ask myself daily "how do you feel", "how do you think you look?" "How do my cloths feel/fit?" Everything else is just a number.

Remember that what matters to you is feeling good and being satisfied. Every single day from the minute you get up until you fall asleep at night you should be having a conversation with your body. "What do you want?" And "how do you feel?" That is it! Your body will tell you when it is hungry or thirsty or needs exercise or has had to much sun. Trust it. Your body tells you everything, so listen carefully and allow it to be fed and happy and relaxed.

Third you are going to have to little by little shift your thinking into believing what I say is true. Food is YOUR friend. Imagine it. Food is here to be enjoyed by you. Can you embrace all food items as friendly and good and to be enjoyed? You have learned that food makes you fat. You are going to have to trust and learn that food is neutral. Food is what you make it. And we can decide right now that it is good. All of it! Yes, truly all of it! Even chocolate. Even sour cream. Even pasta. All food is good for you. There are no bad foods that you have to deny yourself of partaking in.

And finally, yet most important, you will need to learn to

Embrace yourself right where you are at. Love your body and yourself. Go look in the mirror and look in your eyes and ask "what do you think about me?" And really look deeply into your own eyes. You will hear no other response other than I love you. I adore you. If you don't hear that then you are not listening or your mind is getting in the way because your own inner being adores you. And once you are done looking within, look around to help you be reminded that you are so fortunate and it could always be worse. There is always someone else who has it worse than we do. Embrace all of the positives in your life, with your health, and with your body. Count your blessings. Do you maybe need to only lose 15-20 pounds? like I did? How fortunate for you. You don't have to lose 50 like perhaps the next person reading this ebook does. And even if it is 50 or 200, the weight is not the issue. Not anymore! We have taken our eyes off of the weight and off of the food and we have now drawn our attention to ourselves. Who am I? What do I want? How do I feel?

What am I willing to do to get and have what I want? What you focus on expands and it is not going to be a thick waistline any more. Loving yourself and loving food. What we focus on expands. So we have determined that food is neutral and we eat when we are hungry. We ask our bodies what it wants and we allow it to be fed and satisfied. No more fear of food or failing at diets or punishing ourselves. Find something to enjoy today about your body and give thanks. Maybe it is that is gets you from place to place and you can take lovely walks every day. Maybe you still love to dance and feel rather sensual as you let your body move. Feel good right now in your body and rejoice! And then go enjoy a great meal!

It took me eight years to figure this out, but the weight is off and I look and feel great. I am my ideal weight and size. I have kept it off for 11 years, without ever turning back. It has been effortless. Food is my friend and is a pleasure that I enjoy daily. My body is my friend, which I am so grateful for and it tells me everything I need to know about how to look and feel great. I have never been so unencumbered by extra rules that were just clogging my mind and taking up my energy. Be "weightless" in that extra "baggage" department.

Chapter 3

Through The Fear and Into The Frying Pan

"Befriending your body is the only way we know of
coming to understand that your body is resilient and that it
knows what to do, and that it will be whatever you ask it to
be. But you have to ask it to be that in a place of
nonresistance. It's the most significant information
that we have ever expressed relative to your physical body
and food. You must love your body, and then lovingly give
it the food. And when you love your body and lovingly
give it the food, it matters not what food you give it."
>From Abraham-Hicks Workshop
Asheville, NC -- 10/29/00

Facing your fears. You might be saying but what if I allow myself to eat all of these thing? Won't I gain weight? No, you are not going to gain weight. You will lose weight. Here's why: First of all when you aren't feeding your body, and you are living on lettuce everyday your metabolism drops. When your metabolism drops your body holds onto and wants to store the fat. It reaches a set point and that is why so many dieters complain of reaching a plateau and not being able to lose weight even when they are consuming so few calories. Increasing your calorie intake also increases your metabolism which in turn tells your body it doesn't have to panic and hold onto its fat or weight any longer. Rule #1. Eating is good. Starving is bad. Also, let's just say that we let you go nuts! No holds barred! Eat any and everything you want and as much of it as you like. And let's say you did. Now, if you haven't had any Doritos for the last six months, and no pie for the last three months I would not blame you if you went a little over board at first.

If you haven't had a piece of pizza in a while you might feel like eating the whole pizza. No one really craves chocolate or pizza so much that they would want to eat it all day long and for each meal. It would make you sick! And if you are saying "oh yeah, I could eat chocolate and Only chocolate for every meal". Then my guess is that you have been very deprived and you need to let yourself go eat chocolate. Sooner than later, your body will be saying it wants something else. After I have let myself splurge on a hot fudge sundae, I want a fresh lettuce salad with cold cucumbers slices and cherry tomatoes. I crave it. Most weight issues are caused by feeling deprived and so we binge, or feeling like we may never get a chance to eat again, or that certain item again, so we do it even if we are full/satisfied. So I recommend giving yourself permission to go for it. Get it out of your system.

And don't beat yourself up if you gain a pound or two. If that is what feels good right now, do it! Give yourself permission and go for it! But my guess is that once you give yourself permission to eat whatever you want, whenever you want you will no longer feel so obsessive about food again. You will be able to embrace it knowing you now sit at the banquet of life and it is yours for the choosing and eating. Your fear is gone. You just walked right through your fear and have emerged transformed. You love food and food loves you. I like to use the word satisfied. I do not like to feel "full". I can usually feel myself begin to start feeling satisfied as I eat a meal, and I begin to slow down before I feel full. I am not afraid to leave food on my plate. As a matter a fact I usually take too much food. It all looks so good and I want a little bit of everything. But if I take a small scoop of everything, like a bite size of everything it would look silly, so I always take too much.

When you aren't depriving yourself, it takes no effort at all to eat just one. I now can eat a bowl or ice cream and not have to eat a whole carton. I can have a handful of M&M's and not have to eat the whole bag.

What freedom!

Chapter 4

Grazing

"Variety is the soul of pleasure."
Aphra Behn

The key here is to remember to let yourself always feel satisfied. No more rules. No more listening to other people, even "experts". Just listen to yourself. If you feel like getting up in the morning and having pizza, have pizza. If you don't have much of an appetite in the morning and you finally remember to eat at 2 p.m. that is ok too. You don't have to eat breakfast as some dietitians would say. Another "rule" I never follow is not eating before bedtime. If you are hungry at 9 p.m., and haven't eaten for a while, make sure you have something in your stomach so that you are not up at 3 a.m. starving.

I am a grazer. I must eat 5-6 small meals every day. By eating many small meals each day my stomach shrinks. Therefore I get full faster. You will not be able to eat a large 5 coarse meal ever again. You will sit down to Thanksgiving now with complete and utter freedom to eat whatever you like. But make sure you eat dessert first, because you will be full after having eaten a bite of every delicious dish on the table. And remember it is okay to leave food on your plate. My grandmother always said that leaving food on your plate was good etiquette. Then again, my parents told me that there were starving children in China and I should clean my plate. Even if there are starving children down the block, unless you are going to walk your plate over to their residence it is not going to do them any good. In other words, you over eating does not benefit anyone. Just throw the extra food on your plate away. Or give it to the dog.

There is a thin person within you. Just look at yourself as Another Michael Angelo. Now your only job is to find that vision of your thin self in your minds eye and begin sculpting, shaping, and forming your body to fit that vision.

Chapter 5

Keep It Simple

"I like nonsense, it wakes up the brain cells. Fantasy is a necessary ingredient in living. It is a way of looking at life through the wrong end of the telescope. Which is what I do. And that enables you to laugh at life's' realities."
Dr. Seuss

Now that you've befriended food and embraced your body just as it is, and you have thrown away your scales and diet books, you are ready for the good stuff. You are probably wondering if there isn't more to it than this. What is the catch? No catch. However you are going to have to let go of one more thing.

This is so simple that you may think is sounds nonsensical. But believe me this works. It has worked for many people and it can work for you! This is the most effective weight control plan I have ever been on. Here goes. I am going to ask you to do some closet cleaning. Find all of the sweat pants and stretch pants that you can find and gather them and box them up. Now take them and give them to someone less fortunate than yourself. No cheating! You cannot hang onto another pair of lounging pants! They all have to go. And those bib-overalls too. If you have any "moo-moos" as my mom would call them, or slip on tent dresses, those will need to be included in the box that is going to the Salvation Army.

Kiss them good-bye and thank them for all of the comfort And relaxation they gave you, because they are a part of your past. Over the years as you have over eaten, the other way that you have lost touch with your body and how you feel is that you have allowed it to expand by buying bigger sizes of cloths each time your wardrobe got snug. Your body was saying "time to cut back", and you said; "no that is too hard. I will just go buy a new pair of bigger pants." Right? And then after work when you get home you unwind and throw on some sweat pants before dinner. And then after dinner you sit around and if you feel like a snack you have one later and this all feels great! You have told your body "see this elastic waist band? It stretches. And if you would like to expand into it you can." And your body has willingly to comply. Now onto your future and how we are going to change that.

Now I want you to go back to your closets and drawers and dig out all of your jeans and slacks and corduroys. Any fitted pant items. Isn't this fun?

Now look at them all.

How many different sizes do you own right now in your closet? One or two? Three or four? Now line them up from largest (most recent) to smallest (those you absolutely love and can't wait to get back into.) First of all I want you to put on your familiar jeans that you wear daily at present. Try them on and look in the mirror and see how they fit. Feel how they fit. Do you like the way they feel and fit? Do you like the way you look and feel? Would you like it to be different? Better? Would you like to fit into the next smallest size down and then the next until you are finally wearing the ones you adore and can't wait to get into? Of coarse you do! If they are still in your closet then you still have a dream and a vision of seeing yourself wearing those exact jeans. Good for you. You still believe in yourself. You know deep down that there is a thinner person in you just longing to get out. Excellent! Now hold that thought! This is what you want. This is what you will have. It can be done, and sooner than you think!

Here is what you do.

The next step is to try on the next pair of pants, just down one size from the ones you have on. You know the ones you had on two days ago or last week but retired them because they were too snug? Yeah, those are the ones. Or perhaps they are the ones deep in the back of your closet that you haven't dug out for a year or so. Again, good for you. This means you have maintained the same weight for quite a while without gaining more. So you know it can be done. You have proven to yourself that you can set a weight point and hold it steady long term. You just want to set it lower now. So, take a deep breath and relax and try on those jeans now. I know they are going to be snug and feel uncomfortable. Really uncomfortable for awhile. But just do it. If you have to lay on your bed and suck it in a little to get them zipped up, go ahead and do that. Now this is not supposed to be painful. If you don't have a pair of jeans that are just a size too small, perhaps go to the used clothing store and buy a pair since you won't be wearing them long. We want this to be just a little snug. Perhaps a bit uncomfortable. But not painful. Now you can find a long shirt to cover the embarrassing lumps or bumps. But commit to wearing these pants for the next 3 to 7 days. That is it. I promise you if you just commit to wearing these pants to every meal and all day long, you will have lost enough weight to fit comfortably into those jeans. They will then feel like the first pair you put on. The ones you are currently comfortable in. Now you are going to see and feel results fast! With these jeans on today, when you go to McDonalds to eat whatever you want, your tummy is going to tell you exactly what it feels like eating and these jeans are going to help tell your body exactly what it needs. Trust me. You can now eat whatever you want and your body will be giving you new messages. Today you might want to eat only lettuce. But if it does it is not doing it because it has to. Plus you know that tomorrow you will feel differently than today. I guarantee that if you make a promise to yourself to keep these jeans on all day long until you retire and do this for 2-3 days you will notice a difference. Within one week these jeans will fit. You will see results! You are giving your body new messages and your body will be giving you new messages. And don't go jumping on the scale after your first week. Those scales should have been given away. Remember? Fitting into a size smaller week by week should be gratification enough for right now. Trust your body. Listen to your body. This is a new dialogue you are engaging in and if you go back to old habits and looking outside yourself for results you are going to get the same results you got before.

"Insanity is doing the same thing over and over and expecting different results."

Next week you are going to put on the next smaller pair of jeans and you are going to gradually and yet efficiently whittle your way down into those jeans that represent your ideal size. So the main focus here is in being in touch with your body. You are telling your body how you want it to look and it is telling you how it feels.

And put on that belt too. Cinch in your waist line and tell your body that you will have a waist line again. If you over eat your body is just telling you that you are going to have to cut back on the gravy for a day or so to get back into them. So keep going. Day after day and week after week until you have hit your goal. Eat what you want by asking your body what it wants when it is wearing tight clothing. You can have anything. You probably just won't be eating as much of it as you will once your cloths fit properly again.

Chapter 6

Babe's Got Blue Jeans On

"Sometimes you have got to let everything go.
Purge yourself. I did that. I had nothing,
but I had my freedom.....
Whatever is bringing you down, get rid of it,
because you'll find that when you're free,
your true creativity, your true self comes out."
Tina Turner

When you are satisfied and your body/tummy says "enough", push yourself away from the table. There will be more of where that came from tomorrow. Never forget that. You now sit at the banquet of life and you can have anything you want to eat. You can eat what you want and lose and maintain weight. Once you are in your smallest ideal size of jeans (which you will be) you will maintain your weight by using these same simple truths. If you go on a cruise and enjoy all of the delicious food that they have (which I recommend that you do) and if your pants that you have been wearing during the trip get too tight, don't panic! Keep your pants on! That is all there is to this. Do not go back to old habits. They are short term comfort fixes that cause long term discomforts. And whatever you do, never buy a bigger size again! If you haven't done so already, please make sure that you get rid of all of those different sizes of jeans that you have no need of them anymore. Again, give them to someone less fortunate than yourself.

Keep paying attention to your body. And just keep asking your body; "does this feel good", and "what do you want?" We both know that tight pants feel horrible, so practice eating until you are satisfied, and push yourself away from the table before you are full.

This is a partnership. You give your body what it wants with lots of enjoyable food and as long as you stop when it says "I've had plenty thank you", your body will give you what you want in return as well. You will look and feel just as your desires knew you could.

All foods are a blessing and your body is your best friend. Eat what you want and keep your pants on! It has worked for me and it can work for you! By now you know it does not matter what the experts say or what I say that count. It is what you say. Just listen. You are very wise.

"Strength is the ability to break a chocolate bar into 4 pieces with your bare hands - and then eat just one of the pieces." Judith Viorst

And remember; keep your jeans on. ;)